BARBITURATES AND OTHER DEPRESSANTS

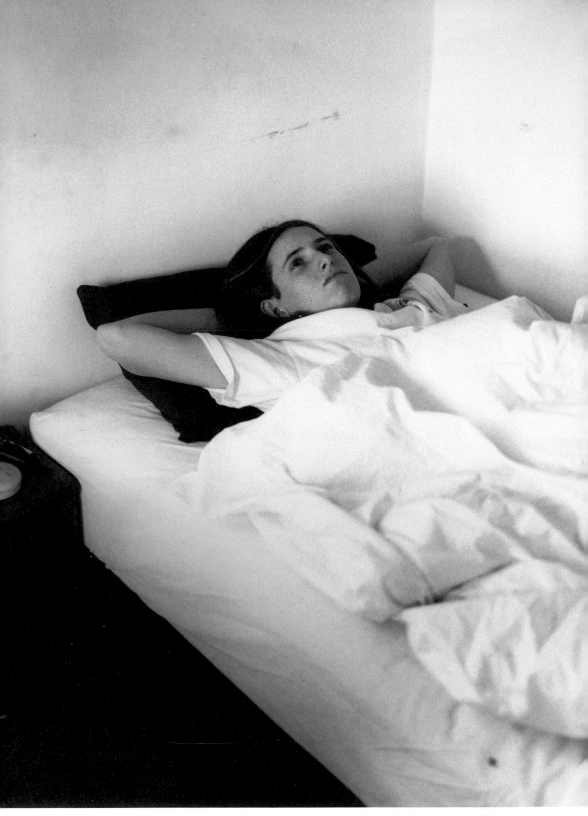

Depressants can change your personality and destroy your life.

THE DRUG ABUSE PREVENTION LIBRARY

BARBITURATES AND OTHER DEPRESSANTS

Lawrence Clayton, Ph.D.

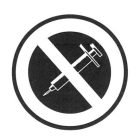

THE ROSEN PUBLISHING GROUP, INC.
NEW YORK

To Gary Cone

The people pictured in this book are only models; they in no way practice or endorse the activities illustrated. Captions serve only to explain the subjects of the photographs and do not imply a connection between real-life models and the staged situations shown. News agency photographs are exceptions.

Published in 1994 by The Rosen Publishing Group, Inc.
29 East 21st Street, New York, NY 10010

First Edition

Printed in Canada

Library of Congress Cataloging-in-Publication Data

Clayton, L. (Lawrence)
    Barbiturates and other depressants / by Lawrence
Clayton.
       p.   cm.—(The Drug abuse prevention library)
       Includes bibliographical references and index.
          ISBN 0-8239-1535-2
          1. Teenagers—Drug use—United States—
          Juvenile literature. 2. Drug abuse—United
          States—Juvenile literature. 3. Barbiturates—
          Juvenile literature. 4. Central nervous system
          depressants—Juvenile literature. [1. Drug abuse.
          2. Barbiturates. 3. Alcoholism.] I. Title.
          II. Series.
          HV5824.Y68C59 1994
          362.29'9—dc20   93-46270
                                          CIP
                                          AC

Contents

14.04

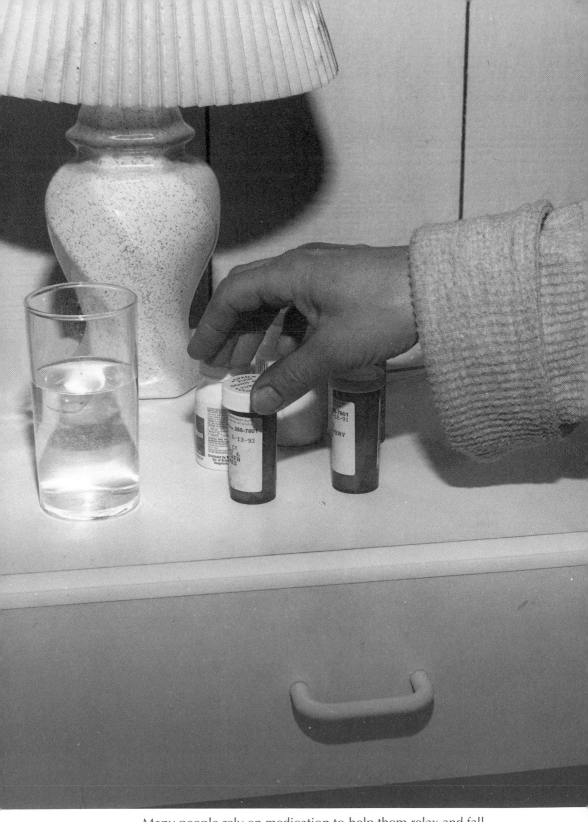

Many people rely on medication to help them relax and fall asleep.

CHAPTER 1

A History of Depressants

*D*epressants are the oldest of all the mood-altering drugs. The records of ancient civilization mention two depressants, opium and alcohol. These drugs are so old that no one is really sure when they were first used. Opium and alcohol, and drugs made from them, were the only depressants for over 4,500 years. Then, in 1838, a new depressant was developed. That started a chain reaction in which thousands of other depressants, each more deadly and more addictive, were developed. Here are some amazing facts about depressants:

- Depressants do have some medical value. Every one of them is useful in treating certain medical problems.

8

- All depressants are addictive.
- In the past, each time a depressant was found to be addictive, another depressant was produced that was believed not to be addictive.
- People welcomed the new, "nonaddictive" drug, and more people used it than had used the other drug.
- Each new depressant was eventually found to be more addictive than the one it replaced.

Depressants have always been the most abused drugs in history. Today, more people are addicted to depressants than ever before. Depressants kill more people and put more in hospitals than any other class of drug.

Each of the depressants has its own unique history. Each has played a part in humankind's ever-widening circle of drug abuse and drug addiction.

Opium

Opium is the oldest known drug of abuse. An ancient people called Sumerians used opium to control pain and anxiety around 3000 B.C. That's almost 5,000 years ago.

The ancient Egyptians used opium for the same purposes around 2000 B.C. They also used it to control headaches and for "female troubles."

It was during the time of the ancient Greeks (1000–338 B.C.) that opium became popular. Doctors prescribed opium to treat almost everything imaginable. They recommended it for pain, anxiety, headache, and female troubles, and also for asthma, cough, stroke, epilepsy, dizziness, and depression.

Soon doctors began reporting that their patients had trouble stopping the use of opium. This caused doctors to worry about its possible harmful effects.

In 1438, a drug called laudanum was made from opium. It was believed not to be addictive. Doctors were pleased with the new drug and began prescribing it for their patients. Within a few years, many thousands of people were addicted to laudanum.

Another depressant made from opium, morphine, was produced in 1808. Doctors immediately began prescribing it in place of laudanum. It, too, was thought to be nonaddictive, but it was hundreds of times more addictive than laudanum.

The hypodermic needle was invented in 1853. This permitted doctors to inject morphine directly into a vein and made it

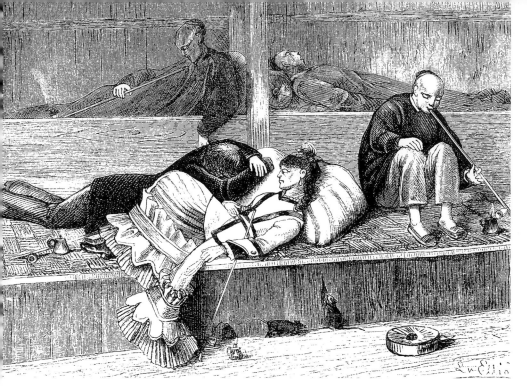

During the nineteenth century, the public often went to opium dens for recreational drug use.

easy to use. Doctors prescribed it to help people addicted to laudanum or alcohol. As a result, thousands of laudanum addicts and alcoholics became morphine addicts. During the American Civil War, so many soldiers on both sides were treated with morphine that the addiction became known as "soldier's disease."

Codeine was the next depressant produced. It was widely prescribed for the ailments treated with morphine, plus colic and teething. As a result, many people—including children—became addicted to codeine. Some were addicted to both codeine and morphine.

In 1898, another depressant made from

opium was introduced that was supposed

to "end morphine addiction forever." It was considered to be "the savior of mankind." Newspaper articles called it the "hero drug." The Bayer company, which produced and sold it, called it heroin. It was 30 times more powerful than morphine, and at least 10 times as addictive.

Finally, the Harrison Narcotics Act of 1914 controlled opium and depressants made from it. Doctors and drug companies were ordered to control narcotics strictly. This mandate, however, caused companies to develop many new kinds of depressants. Some were synthetic (human-made), opium-like drugs. Others were called tranquilizers and barbiturates. The results were deadly. In less than 60 years, thousands of new depressants were introduced, and millions more people became addicted.

Alcohol

Along with narcotics, beer and wine have been used for at least 4,500 years in the Orient, Africa, and Europe. Ancient Chinese, Egyptian, Greek, and Roman doctors prescribed them to help people relax and for sleeplessness.

In many places during that time, the water was not good to drink. The people

12 often drank beer or wine instead. Partly because of this, the use of alcoholic beverages became a common practice.

Almost from the beginning, some people had problems with alcohol. They drank too much, became ill, and passed out. Some became violent, hurting others or themselves. Fathers quit working, and mothers failed to care for their children. Soon leaders in Europe and the Middle East started warning people to be careful about alcohol use.

In the year 494 A.D., people in the Middle East discovered how to make purer forms of alcohol. They called the process *distilling*. Until then, alcoholic drinks were very weak. Beer contained about 6 percent alcohol, and wine about 16 percent. Distilling made it possible for liquors to contain up to 50 percent alcohol. These new, stronger drinks were called brandy, whiskey, gin, rum, and vodka. They, too, were prescribed by doctors.

When people began to settle in the United States, they brought strong liquor with them. It was easy to carry and was widely used for pain and nervousness. Alcoholism was a major problem for the colonists, and it soon became a problem for the Native Americans (Indians) as well.

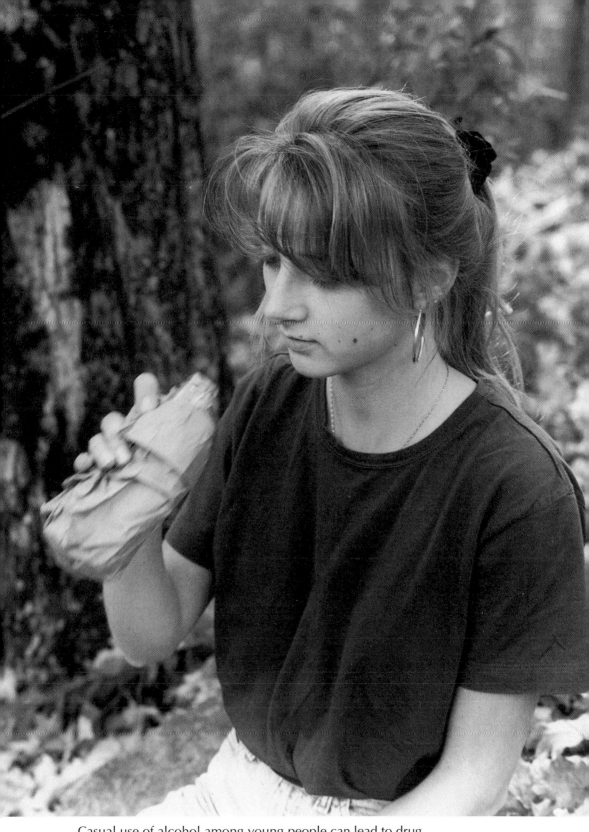

Casual use of alcohol among young people can lead to drug abuse and addiction.

14   In 1919, the United States Congress passed a law forbidding the making, owning, or drinking of alcohol. The law was popularly called Prohibition. Immediately, people began to make it illegally. These people, called bootleggers, had little or no experience making alcohol. Some of the alcohol they made caused people to go blind or die. Criminals banded together in groups that became known as "organized crime syndicates" or "the Mob." (Years later, these organizations turned to distributing and selling drugs.) Criminals like Al Capone made millions of dollars selling bootleg whiskey. The Congress voted to repeal Prohibition in 1933.

Today, alcohol is still the most abused of all the depressants. It is also thought to be the most dangerous. It causes over 500 deaths every day in the United States alone. It has also been shown to be a gateway drug, leading teens to other kinds of drugs. Kids are using it at younger ages and being hurt worse. More teenagers abuse alcohol than any other drug.

Barbiturates

Barbiturates are the second most abused depressant. They were discovered in 1864 when a chemist combined animal urine

and acid from apples. The result was bar- |
bituric acid. In 1903, it was found that
barbiturates were useful in sleeplessness.

Since then, over 2,700 depressants have
been made from barbituric acid. These
barbiturates have proved successful in the
treatment of anxiety, muscular tension,
and pain. They represent about 25 percent
of prescriptions for mood-altering drugs
written by doctors in the United States.

Barbiturates are very dangerous. Like
all depressants, they are basically a poison.
A small dose slows the user's body and
mind. A large dose kills. Barbiturates are
used in suicides more than any other drug.
Many alcohol and drug counselors say,
"There is only one difference between a
drug and a poison, and that's the dose!"

Most people need medical help to with-
draw safely from barbiturate addiction.
Seizures and comas are serious risks. Each
year, about 60 percent of those addicts
who don't seek help to stop, die as a result.

Tranquilizers
Tranquilizers are classed as major and
minor. The major tranquilizers were first
discovered in 1882, but it wasn't until 1952
that they were found to help in lowering
blood pressure.

16   Two years later, tranquilizers were first used in treating the severely mentally ill. Previously, such people were confined in mental hospitals, some for the rest of their lives. The major tranquilizers have made it possible for many people with mental illness to remain with their families and to live productive lives.

The minor tranquilizers were discovered in 1955. Like barbiturates, they were found helpful in treating anxiety and sleeplessness and as muscle relaxers.

The first of these depressants was sold as Librium. Doctors thought it would be a wonder drug, as the major tranquilizers had been. They believed that it would do everything barbiturates did but would not be addictive. After prescribing it for hundreds of thousands of patients, doctors discovered that many people *had* become addicted. This caused a great deal of disappointment and concern.

It also caused a lot of research. Finally, a new tranquilizer was developed, Valium. It worked as well as Librium, and it was thought to be nonaddictive. Valium became the wonder drug of the 1960s. It was prescribed for millions of patients, especially housewives. It was even called "mother's little helper" in a popular

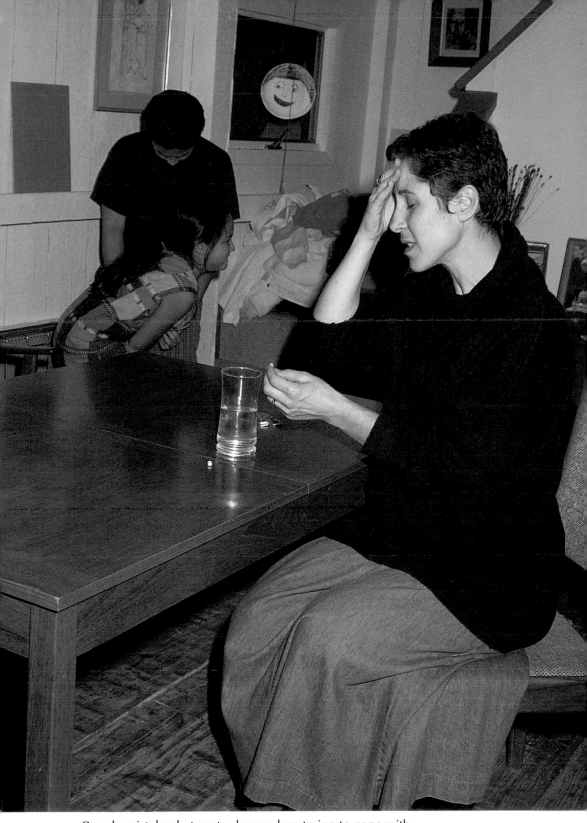

People mistakenly turn to drugs when trying to cope with the stress of daily life.

18 Beatles' song. By the early 1970s, more people were addicted to Valium than had been addicted to Librium.

Next, the tranquilizer Xanax was developed. Many times more powerful than Valium, it, too, was thought to be nonaddictive. Once again, it was prescribed for millions of patients, and once again, people became addicted. Within four years of its appearance, Xanax became the most widely prescribed depressant in America. Finally, in 1984, tranquilizers were added to the growing list of severely dangerous substances.

With the introduction of the prescription depressants, a new drug era began. Organized crime became heavily involved in distributing and selling prescription drugs. This made drugs available to every adult, teenager, and child in America. Gradually, a group of users during the 1960s came to be known as "the drug culture." This movement became a major influence on young people. Many of them have joined "drug culture" gangs.

Depressants have played an important part in the spread of drug addiction. Let us take a closer look at what these drugs do, how they are used, and their effects on abusers.

CHAPTER 2

Types of Depressants

It is estimated that over 90 percent of the population of the United States will use a depressant at some time during their lives. Over 60 percent will do so before finishing high school.

All depressants slow down (or depress) the user's mind and body. They slow down the heart and lungs. Too much depressant causes the heart to stop beating and the lungs to quit breathing. When that happens, the user dies.

Because depressants slow the functioning of the brain, abusers think more slowly. They react more slowly. Because of this, it is dangerous for abusers to drive cars or operate equipment. In fact, depressant abuse causes over half of the accidental deaths in the United States.

19

20   Depressants also cause over half of the accidental poisonings. This is because many abusers do not realize that these drugs can have a "multiplying" effect when taken with other depressants. For example, if someone drinks alcohol and takes a barbiturate, the effect may be 10 times stronger than either one taken separately.

Abusers say that depressants make them feel at peace, happy, sexy, friendly, relaxed, uninhibited, confident, fearless, and without pain. Depressants can also cause weight gain. Abusers' slowed down bodies do not burn calories very well.

People who abuse depressants can be identified by slurred speech, staggering, lack of coordination, temporary memory loss, nodding off (falling asleep), pinpoint pupils, laziness, yawning, and lack of motivation.

Depressants are extremely addictive. People who abuse them must constantly increase the amount they use. To do so becomes more and more dangerous with each use. Any depressant will kill if taken in a large enough quantity. So each time abusers increase the amount of drug, the closer they come to the point at which the drug will kill them.

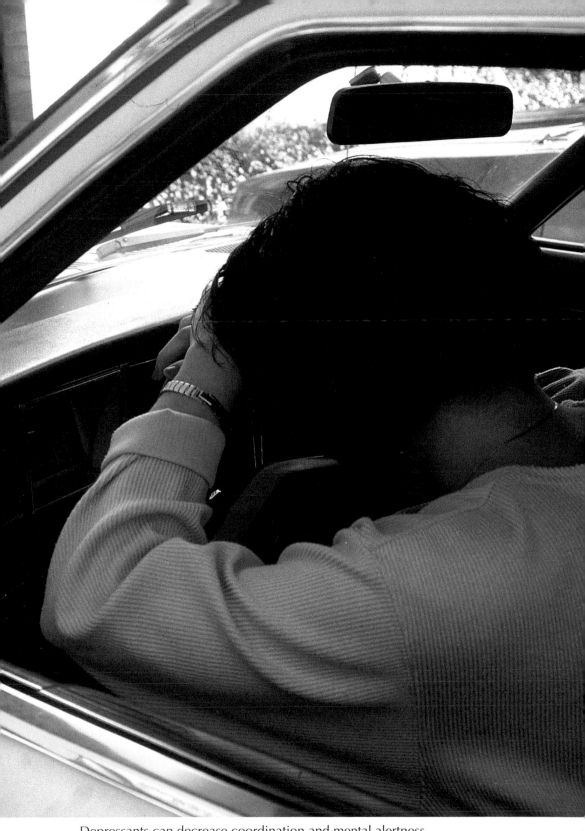

Depressants can decrease coordination and mental alertness.

22 *Withdrawal*

Using depressants can be dangerous, but so can stopping. When abusers try to stop using depressants without a doctor's help (called going "cold turkey"), they may go into withdrawal. This also can kill them. Here is what happens.

Without depressants, withdrawal starts within 12 to 24 hours. Abusers soon begin to feel anxious and have trouble sitting still. After 24 hours, they begin to feel angry and shaky. Withdrawal becomes most severe after 72 hours when the abusers start to feel sick. They may suffer severe stomach cramps and vomit. Their heartbeat speeds up, they become extremely anxious, and they sweat profusely. They become delirious, seeing, hearing, and smelling things that are not real. They may also have convulsions and go into a coma. This is the most serious risk. Of the abusers who become delirious and have convulsions, about half die unless they get medical help.

Narcotics

Narcotics are depressants. Included in this class are opium, drugs made from opium, and synthetic drugs that act like

NARCOTICS (FROM OPIUM)

Medical Term	Scientific Name	Street Name	Medical Uses	Form/Size
Opium	Papaver somniferum	O, Opi	Pain	No longer in general use
Heroin	diaceymeta-morphine	H, Smack	Pain	Powder
Dilaudid	papaverine	Di, Did	Pain	Pills of 1, 2, 3, and 4-mg
Codeine	codeine	Code	Pain Coughs	Syrup
Percodan	oxycodone	Perc	Pain	2.25-, 4.5-, and 5-mg pills
Laudanum	laudanum	None	Pain	No longer in general use
Morphine	morphine, sulphate	M, Big M, Morph	Pain	Liquid

NARCOTICS (HUMAN-MADE)

Medical Term	Scientific Name	Street Name	Medical Uses	Form/Size
Methadone	methadone	Done	Heroin detoxification	Liquid
Sublimaze	fentanyl	Sub, Doc	Pain	Liquid
Demerol	meperidine	Demi	Pain	50- and 100-mg pills
Talwin	pentazocine	Tall	Pain	50-mg pills and liquid
Darvon	propoxyphene hydrochloride	Darv, Vony	Pain	65- and 100-mg pill

24 opium. Drugs made from opium are laudanum, morphine, codeine, Percodan, Dilaudid, and heroin. Synthetic depressants that act like opium are methadone, Demerol, Talwin, Darvon, and Sublimaze.

Alcohol

The scientific name of this depressant is ethyl alcohol or ethanol. All alcohol comes in liquid form. The four basic kinds of alcoholic drinks are beer, wine, cordials, and hard liquor.

Beer is packaged in cans or bottles. It is made from rotting grain. It usually contains about 6 percent alcohol.

Wine is sold in quart, half-gallon, or gallon bottles. It is made from rotting fruit. It usually contains about 12 percent alcohol.

Cordials come in pint or quart bottles. They are made from wine combined with hard liquor. The alcohol content is about 20 percent.

Hard liquor is bottled in several sizes: half-pint, pint, four-fifths of a quart (called "a fifth"), quart, half-gallon, and gallon. It is made from cooking rotted grain or fruit and collecting the alcohol as it evaporates. This makes hard liquor much stronger than beer or wine. It is about 50 percent alcohol. Some of the more common hard liquors are vodka, rum, brandy, gin, and whiskey.

Many people believe that they can become alcoholic only by drinking hard liquor, but this is *not* true. The fact is that about the same amount of alcohol is contained in a can of beer, a glass of wine, and a shot of hard liquor. (A shot is about an ounce, the amount usually found in a mixed drink.) More people are addicted to alcohol than to any other depressant.

Barbiturates

There are more than 2,700 drugs under this heading, more than in any other class of depressants. Barbiturates include all drugs made from barbituric acid.

Barbiturates have several medical uses. They are prescribed for sleeplessness, to prevent seizures, to overcome extreme nervousness, and to treat hyperactivity. They are also effective to relieve pain and relax sore, tense muscles.

Barbiturates usually come in pill or capsule form and are taken by mouth. Some of the major barbiturates are described below.

26   **Amytal**. The scientific name is Amyobarbital. It comes in four small pill sizes: 15-mg, tan; 30-mg, gold; 50-mg, peach colored; and 100-mg, pink. Amytal also comes in a syrup. A form of Amytal with sodium added comes in a light blue capsule, 65-mg or 200-mg.

    Butisol comes in 15- and 30-mg, light blue capsules.

    Carbital comes in 1.25- and 4-grain, clear capsules.

    Fiorinal comes in two 50-mg forms: a large white pill and a large, dark green and lime green capsule. Fiorinal also comes with codeine added in several sizes and colors of capsule.

    Nembutal. The scientific name is pentobarbital. It comes in three capsule sizes: 30-mg, yellow; 50-mg, orange and clear; and 100-mg, yellow. Nembutal also is made in liquid and suppository forms.

    Phenobarbital. The scientific name is pentobarbital sodium. It comes in .25-,.5-, and 1.5-grain, round white pills. It also comes in syrup, liquid, and tubex (inject-able) form.

    Seconal comes in 50- and 100-mg, or-ange capsules.

    Tuinal comes in 50-, 100-, and 200-mg, orange and blue capsules.

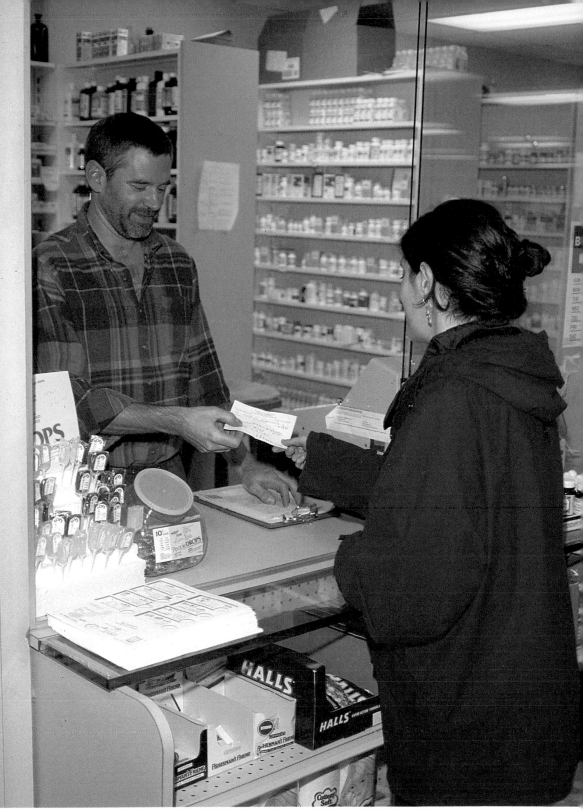

Your pharmacist will be happy to answer questions about
medication prescribed for you by your doctor.

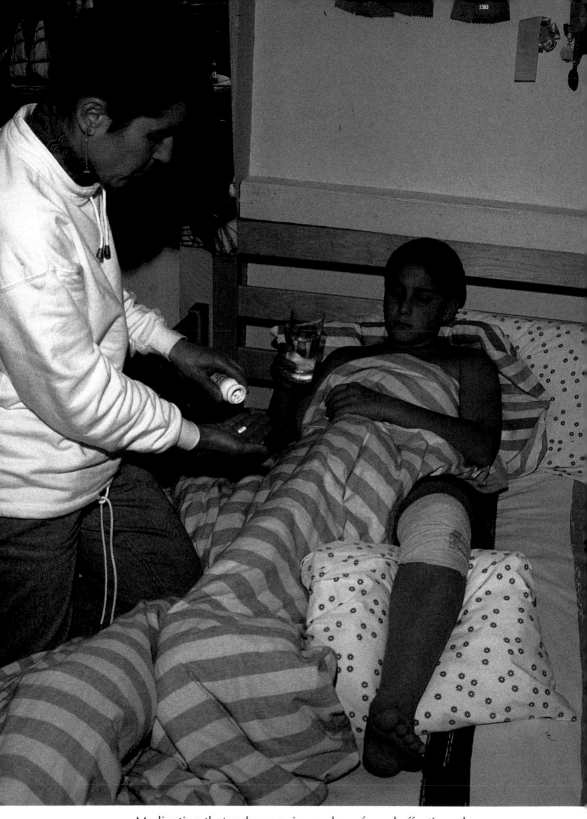

Medication that reduces pain can be safe and effective when taken as directed.

Tranquilizers

Both major and minor tranquilizers are legal drugs.

Some of the major tranquilizers are Mellaril, Thorazine, Phenothiazine, and Compazine. They are primarily used in treating the seriously mentally ill. The drugs are seldom abused— such powerful medication is given under close supervision.

Millions of people, however, have become addicted to the minor tranquilizers. These are used to treat people who are nervous, angry, or have trouble sleeping. Minor tranquilizers are controlled substances. Three of these drugs that are the most often prescribed by doctors are also the most abused.

Librium. The scientific name is chlordiazepoxide. It comes in three capsule sizes: 5-mg, yellow and green; 10-mg, light and dark green; and 25-mg, green and cream colored.

Valium. The scientific name is diazepam. It comes in three sizes of pills: 2-mg, white; 5-mg, yellow; and 10-mg, light blue. It also comes in a liquid form.

Xanax. The scientific name is alprazolam. It comes in four pill sizes: .25-mg, white; .5-mg, peach; 1-mg, purple; and 2-mg, white.

30 | *Other Depressants*

There are several other mood-altering drugs that are chemically different from the barbiturates and the tranquilizers. These depressants are also prescription drugs, legally available only from doctors. Six of these drugs are the most used and abused.

Quaalude. The scientific name is methaqualone. The street name is "ludes." Quaalude is available in two sizes: 150-mg, a medium-sized white pill, and 300-mg, a large white pill.

Placidyl. The scientific name is ethchlorvynol. Street names are "placid" and "the peace pill." It comes in four sizes. The 100-, 200-, and 500-mg sizes are reddish-brown pills filled with clear liquid. The 750-mg size is an extra large dark green capsule containing a clear liquid.

Doriden. The scientific name is glutethimide. It comes in two sizes, but three types: .25-gm, a medium-sized white tablet; and .5-gm, a large white tablet bearing the numbers 354 or a medium-sized, blue and white capsule.

Dalmane. The scientific name is flurazepam hydrochloride. It comes in 15-mg and 30-mg orange and cream colored capsules.

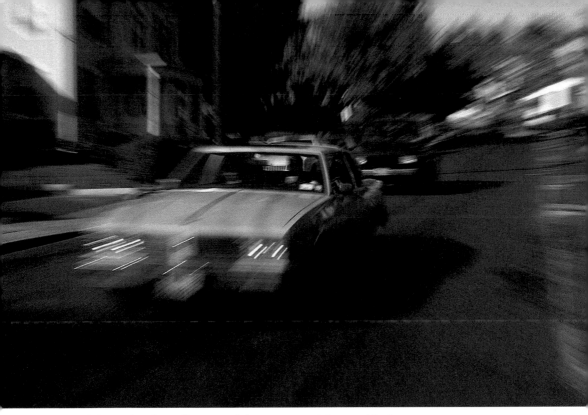

While under the influence of drugs, your vision and judgment may be severely distorted.

Nortec. The scientific name is chloral hydrate. It comes in a 500-mg, lime green or red capsule filled with a clear liquid. It also comes in syrup form.

Ativan. The scientific name is lorazepam. It comes in three sizes: .5 mg, a tiny round white pill; 1-mg, a small, oblong white pill; and 2-mg, a small, foot-ball-shaped pill. It is also available in liquid form.

At this point, you know a lot about the history, medical uses, names, appearance, and abuse problems of depressants. Now it is time to find out how they can change your personality.

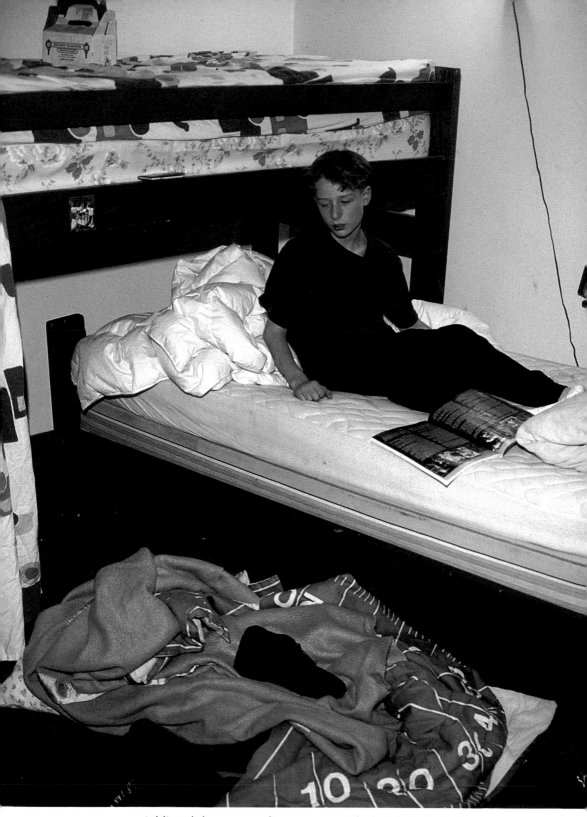

Addicted depressant abusers cannot deal with their feelings in healthy ways. They lose control of their lives.

CHAPTER 3

What Depressants Do to Your Personality

It may be hard to understand, but depressant abuse *will* change your personality. Depressant abusers are in a great deal of emotional pain. It hurts them to give up control of their mind, body, and life. To cope with this pain, abusers usually begin to think and act in unusual ways.

Family members and friends may be the first to notice a change in the depressant abuser. They are often quite upset with the abuser because the changes are both negative and severe.

Alcohol and drug counselors call these changes "the emotional consequences of abuse." This means that those who abuse depressants are paying a mental price for their drug habit. Let's take a closer look at these changes.

34 | *Denial*

Being "in denial" is a way of dealing with emotional pain by believing that the painful event never happened. A person who is in denial really doesn't know that something painful has happened.

Imagine being in a car wreck in which your best friend was killed, then telling yourself that there was no wreck and believing that your friend was still alive. That's exactly what it's like to be in denial.

Depressant abusers often can't understand why people say such terrible things about them. They are unable to see their behavior as others see it.

Phil, age 13

Phil began smoking his older brother's marijuana when he was 10. He started drinking two months later. By the time he was 12, he was using several types of depressants every day.

One day his teacher called his father to ask if Phil was getting enough rest and food at home. She explained that the school had a hot lunch program for kids who couldn't afford to pay. She said that Phil seemed very tired and often fell asleep in class. She was sure that he must be run down.

Phil's father, a wealthy businessman, started looking into the problem. He talked to Phil's friends and their parents. Little by little the story unfolded. Phil was abusing depressants. At first, it was hard for Phil's father to believe, but then he found a bottle of barbiturates in Phil's room.

Phil's father confronted his son. He told his son what the teachers and his friends had said, and showed him the bottle of pills. Phil finally admitted that he was taking drugs but angrily denied falling asleep at school.

At that point, Phil's father took him to a hospital that specialized in barbiturate addiction. Even after months in the hospital, Phil still did not believe that he ever fell asleep at school.

Projection

Projection is another way in which depressant abusers deal with severe emotional pain. They "give" their pain to someone else by believing that it is the other person's pain.

Alcohol and drug counselors believe that of all those who abuse drugs, the depressant abusers are in the most emotional pain. This may explain why so many depressant abusers commit suicide.

36 | *Jenny, age 17*

Jenny began drinking beer when she was 13. A year later, she was taking her mother's sleeping pills. By the time she was 15, she had a serious drug habit. She was addicted to Quaaludes.

One night at a friend's house, Jenny drank several alcoholic drinks. She had already taken her usual amount of Quaaludes. After a while, she began slurring her words and couldn't seem to walk right. Then she announced that she was going home and asked for the keys to her boyfriend's car. He gave them to her, and she staggered out the door.

Parents may be unaware that their own pills pose a threat to an unstable teenage son or daughter.

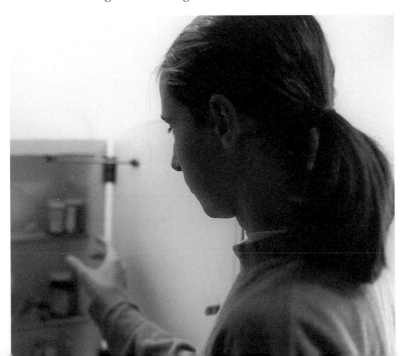

Later, Jenny's friends noticed that the car was still in the driveway. Looking in, they found her slumped over the steering wheel. They couldn't awaken her.

At the hospital, Jenny's stomach was pumped and she was given several kinds of medication. Nothing seemed to help. She was in a coma for three weeks. The doctor told her family that she might never wake up. Then one day she just opened her eyes, sat up, and tried to talk. She had survived.

After several days and many tests, however, the doctor told Jenny and her family that she would never be able to talk again. The speech center of her brain had been too badly damaged.

That didn't seem to bother Jenny at all. Later she wrote a note and handed it to a nurse. The note said, "I don't know why, but my mom is really upset about this speech thing. Can you help her?"

Minimizing

Minimizing is a way for an abuser to hide painful information from him or herself. He or she plays down the facts. The abuser may not understand how strange his or her behavior has become nor what all the fuss is about.

38 　　Most alcohol and drug counselors wait until friends and family members are present before asking how much alcohol or drugs the abuser uses. Abusers minimize to such an extent that they can't be trusted to know their level of use.

Jack, age 15

Jack began taking Quaaludes when he was 12. He never thought that he could become addicted to them. He just liked how they made him feel. Within a year, he was taking several pills a day. He had also become very quiet, was failing several classes, and had put on a lot of weight.

One day, Jack's mother discovered some pills in his room. She didn't recognize them, so she took them to a pharmacist. He told her that the medication could be dangerous and addicting.

When Jack got home that evening, his mother demanded that he tell her the truth, and he did. At least, he told her as much as he knew. He said that he had been using Quaaludes for three months and that he only used one or two a week.

Several days later, one of Jack's friends was caught selling drugs. During questioning, he revealed that Jack was his biggest customer.

Jack's mother was truly shocked to find out that Jack was using 10 times as much as he had told her. Alarmed, she put him in a hospital for drug treatment. Later, his doctor said he was amazed that Jack was still alive.

Blaming
Blaming is still another way abusers deal with the emotional pain of addiction. They simply blame their problems on someone else—often someone who cares about them.

Amy, age 10
Amy's mother worried about almost everything. Most of all, she worried that she wouldn't be a good mother to Amy. Amy's father had died three years earlier, and her mother was having a tough time managing without him. Her doctor had put her on tranquilizers.

Amy was also in pain because of her father's death. She overheard her mother telling a friend that certain pills she had really helped. That evening Amy took one of her mother's pills. Soon she was feeling a lot better. Taking her mother's medicine became a habit. By the time she was nine, Amy was an addict.

40   The doctor finally became suspicious when her mother called to ask for another refill. "Mrs. Johnson," he said, "I am afraid you are taking way too much." After questioning her, he asked, "Well, if you say you're not taking them, who is?" Later that day, Amy's mother saw Amy poking around in the medicine cabinet. She asked firmly, "Amy, have you been taking my medicine?" Amy screamed, "If you weren't such a rotten mother, I wouldn't need to take your pills!"

Repression of Feelings

Almost all depressant abusers respond to the emotional pain of addiction by repressing (not dealing with) their feelings. They repress even the good feelings, because they are afraid to feel anything.

This causes them to be very robot-like. They deal with facts, but avoid feelings. That causes abusers even more pain, because most people find it difficult to relate to others who show no feelings.

Lorenzo, age 22

Lorenzo had used depressants since he was 12. He started drinking wine with his father. By the time he was 16, he would use any depressant he could find—beer, whiskey, barbiturates, narcotics.

Dolores had known Lorenzo most of her life. Their parents had come from Mexico together and had always been close. Dolores and Lorenzo had been going together for six years. Dolores wanted to get married. But Lorenzo acted as if he didn't care about anything.

The local priest knew the couple well. Fortunately, he also understood alcohol and drugs. He recognized Lorenzo's problem. He put Lorenzo in touch with a counselor who specialized in treating depressant addiction.

Now Lorenzo and Dolores are married. Lorenzo has a good job, and Dolores is expecting a child. "The best thing," said Lorenzo, "is that I can feel again."

Expression of Anger

Depressant abusers tend to be angry most of the time. Anger may be the only feeling that they express. When they are running low on drugs or are in withdrawal, some depressant abusers become violent. Others can be abusive at any time.

It is important to remember that the anger from depressant abuse can be very

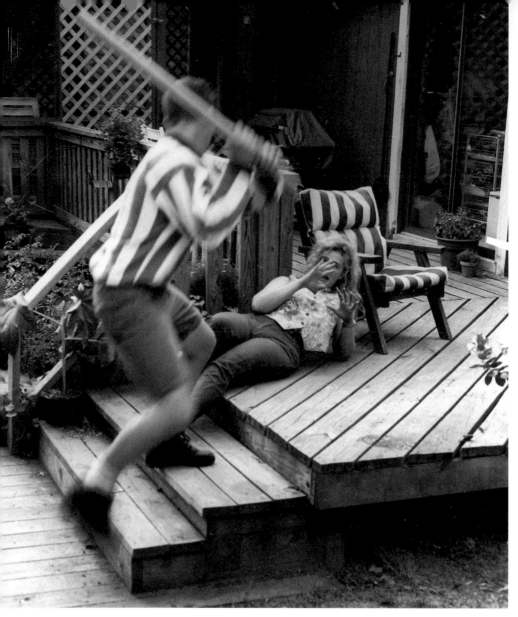

Even family members are not safe when the depressant abuser becomes violent.

dangerous. In fact, depressant abuse plays a part in more than half of all family violence (including murders). Dr. George Viallant of Dartmouth Medical School describes depressant abuse as "the only illness which causes its victims to be overly angry at the people they most love."

Jan, age 16

Jan started drinking when she was 11. By the time she was 13, she had begun using barbiturates, but she still drank alcohol when she couldn't get barbiturates. Sometimes she used them at the same time.

One day her little brother, Larry, said, "I really like that outfit you have on." Jan screamed at him, "You're such a dweeb. How would you know what looks good?" Larry said, "Well, *excuse me!*" Jan grabbed an ashtray and threw it at him, hitting him in the corner of the eye.

It took 48 stitches to close the wound. Her mother asked Jan why she had done such a terrible thing. Jan shouted, "Why are you always picking on me? If he had kept his stupid mouth shut, none of this would have happened!"

Blackouts

Almost all depressant abusers have blackouts. They can't remember what they did or said, or where they were. It's as if their memory had been erased. This can be frightening to abusers and to their family and friends. It can also be confusing.

Confabulation is a word for the way depressant abusers deal with not being able to remember. Their mind simply "fills in

44 the blanks" by making up a version of what happened. People who were with them know exactly what happened. Then, when they hear the abuser saying something entirely different, they get confused. At first, they think that the abuser is just lying. They are amazed to discover that the person actually believes the made-up story.

Cathy, age 14

Cathy's father was an alcoholic. One evening, he came home drunk and beat Cathy's mother. He kicked several holes in the wall, broke up furniture, and shot a hole in the television set. Finally, he stumbled off to bed.

The next morning, he punished Cathy for damaging the house. He was very angry, and said, "Don't bring those friends of yours to this house again! Next time, I'll have them all put in jail!"

This really confused and angered Cathy at first. But she finally realized that her father believed what he said. When she tried to explain that he had actually been at fault, he started yelling at her, saying, "No daughter of mine is going to get away with lying like that!"

Paranoia

The word "paranoia" means unreasonable fear. Depressant abusers are usually afraid of many reasonable things. They are afraid they'll be caught. They are afraid they will run out of drugs. They are afraid they can't trust their friends. But aside from the reasonable fears, many abusers come to fear almost everything.

Sheena, age 16

No one would have guessed that Sheena had problems with fear. She had always been an especially confident person. She was a cheerleader and captain of the girls' volleyball team.

At 14, Sheena had started using barbiturates. Within a year, she was addicted. She was convinced that she played better, cheered better, and looked better when she was high. One day some friends found her hiding under a bridge, screaming, "Don't let them get me! Don't tell them where I am, or they will hurt me."

No one is really sure what happened to Sheena. Maybe she got some bad drugs, or maybe she just damaged her brain by using depressants for so long. In any case, Sheena wound up in a mental hospital.

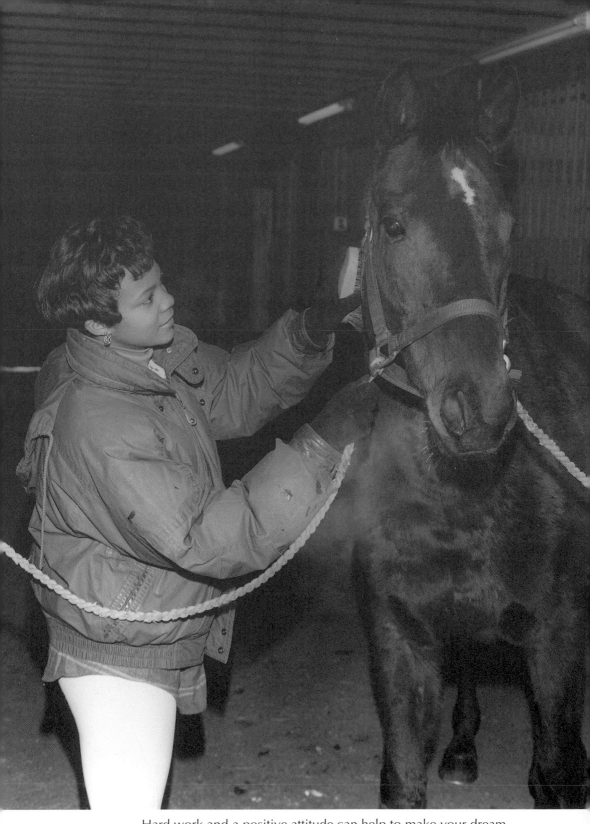

Hard work and a positive attitude can help to make your dream come true.

CHAPTER 4

It's Your Future!

*T*he opening words of the hit motion picture "Pretty Woman" are the same as its closing lines: "What's your dream? Everybody has a dream! This is Hollywood! So, what's your dream?" What's yours?

Counselors tell us that most teenagers have some idea what they want for their future. They may not have all the details worked out, but they have a general idea. Counselors call this the "adolescent life dream."

What is your life dream? Would you like to be really good at something? Would you like to be the best? To be famous? Would you like to have a lot of money? Would you like to do something no one has ever done?

48   No one can say for certain if your dream will come true. But there are some things you can do to increase your chances of making it come true. And if you do these things, your life will be better, even if all of your dream doesn't come true.

Be Willing to Work Hard

There is no substitute for hard work. Ask anyone who ever did something great. They will tell you that it took hard work. Do you want to be a professional basketball star? If you were to ask Michael Jordan, Patrick Ewing, or Charles Barkley, they would tell you that it took years of training. Want to be a great singer? Ask Hammer, Brian Adams, or Garth Brooks. They would tell you the same thing!

It is that way in every field—teaching, sports, the military, politics, writing. If you want to succeed, you have to put in many hours of hard work.

Using depressants can destroy your ability to work hard. Tranquilizers and barbiturates destroy the desire to do anything. Alcohol and narcotics leave you with a depression so severe that you may not even be able to relate to others. For some people, this damage is permanent.

Sun, age 15

Sun's father had always said, "If you want to get anywhere in your life, you must work hard." Sun believed his father. He had dreamed of being a jockey most of his life. He went to the track every day. After getting to know him, the trainers had started to let him exercise the horses. He was becoming a good rider.

Then Sun's cousin introduced him to drinking. Soon, Sun just didn't feel like going to the track. His father was worried, and asked what was wrong. Sun replied, "Nothing." But he continued to drink.

One day, Sun was so drunk that he fell off a horse. The horse was frightened and bolted into the fence, injuring its leg. The trainer said, "Boy, you can ruin your life if you want to, but you aren't going to ruin my horses! You're not riding here again."

Faced with this disgrace, Sun quit drinking altogether. But he became so depressed that he could do nothing but sit and stare. Depressants had taken Sun's desire from him.

Be Determined

Most successful people were very stubborn about pursuing their goals. They reached their goals by putting their dreams first.

50 You can succeed in the same way. If you want to be a great clarinet player, you must be willing to practice while your friends are having fun. If you want to be a great weight lifter, you have to be faithful to a strict workout program, eat right, and get enough sleep.

People who reach their goals are determined. They are totally dedicated to the belief that they will succeed. They don't get distracted by other things.

One of the surest ways to fail is to start abusing depressants. Abusers spend so much time and energy thinking about drugs, and how and where to get them, that they lose sight of their goals.

Sharon, age 16

Sharon wanted to be a mother more than anything. All she thought about was finishing high school, getting married, and having children. No career for her. She was going to be a homemaker and "be there" for her children.

Then she met Jeff. He was addicted to heroin, but Sharon was so much in love that she married him thinking that she could help him. Sometimes she used heroin herself, just because Jeff wanted her to get stoned with him.

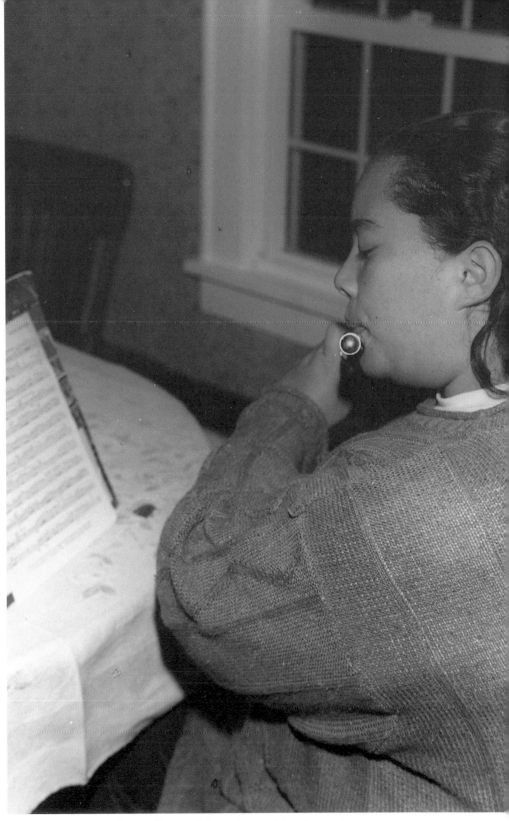

Avoid drugs altogether. Fill your life with activities that make
you feel good about yourself.

52 Sharon dreamed of having children. Today, a part of her dream has come true. She did have a baby. But things are not what she expected. Her husband is usually too stoned to work, and her baby has so many health needs that she must work two jobs to pay the medical bills.

Sharon spends most of her time at the laundromat, the grocery store, or at the kitchen table worrying about their bills. Even if she doesn't get high with Jeff, her dream of "being there" for her children is lost.

Being determined is important. It can be the difference in achieving or not achieving your dream. Abusing depressants can ruin your determination.

Be Sober

Alcohol may damage your abilities so slowly that you hardly notice. Too late, you may realize what has happened to you.

First, depressants make you feel good. Next, they make you believe that you can control them. Then they make you think they aren't hurting you. In the end, they make you believe that nothing else matters. Finally, you discover that they are controlling you.

William, age 18

William had promised himself that he would never abuse alcohol. He hated alcohol. His father had been an alcoholic who had drunk himself to death when William was 12.

William wanted to be a dentist, like his dad. He wanted to have a family, like his dad, but he wanted to live long enough to help his children.

William knew that there was a chance he had inherited his father's tendency to alcoholism. That was why he had promised himself never to use any drugs. Friends had tried to get him to drink, but each time he said, "No way!"

In his senior year of high school, William got a letter from his favorite college. "Congratulations! The faculty and staff at Texas Wesleyan College are proud to inform you that you have been awarded a full-tuition scholarship..." William ran to his mother, shouting, "Mom! I got it! I got it!" His mother hugged him, saying, "I'm proud of you, Son!" Then she began to cry.

You can see your dream come true, just like William. Staying away from alcohol allowed him to make better life choices. Being sober is a big step in making good things happen.

54 | *Believe in Yourself*

You need to have a positive attitude. If you don't believe in yourself, no one else will! Be confident. Believe that you can make your dream happen.

You will have a hard time believing in yourself if you start abusing depressants. Few things can wreck your self-esteem faster than getting hooked on depressants.

Charla, age 17

Charla wanted to be an actress. She had been in all the school plays. Everyone, including her drama coach, said that she had what it took to make it in Hollywood. But all that was before she started abusing Xanax.

Charla had been using the antianxiety drug for over two years. She had tried to quit hundreds of times. Each time she failed she got more depressed, and each time she felt worse about herself. She finally decided it was time to see a doctor for help.

The doctor put Charla in the hospital and got her involved in counseling. He also sent her to a Narcotics Anonymous group. Little by little, Charla learned how to deal with her desire for drugs. And best of all, she began to like herself again.

CHAPTER 5

Getting Help

*O*f all drugs, depressants are the most dangerous to stop using without medical help. Thousands of people die each year trying to quit. If you have been using depressants for a long time, you'll probably need help. Here are some of the people you can turn to.

Your Parents

Some teenagers don't think of their parents as people who could help. Most parents are especially good helpers when given the chance. Your parents may be shocked to learn that you are abusing drugs, but they'll get over it. You might start by giving them this book to read.

56

Your Teacher

Helping young people is part of the reason teachers become teachers. If your teacher doesn't know exactly what to do, he or she usually knows where to find out. So, ask!

Your School Counselor

Counselors are specially trained to help students. Many of them know about drugs. And they also know the kinds of services available in the community.

Your Religious Leader

Many clergypersons understand addiction and know exactly where to refer you. If they have known your family for a long time, they may be extremely helpful when you tell your parents about your drug problem.

Crisis, Drug, and Hot Lines

In larger cities, telephone counseling services are established for the purpose of helping youth. They are staffed by people who understand alcohol and other drugs and know where the best services are.

Some of these services are staffed by peer counselors, people your age who have been trained to help others.

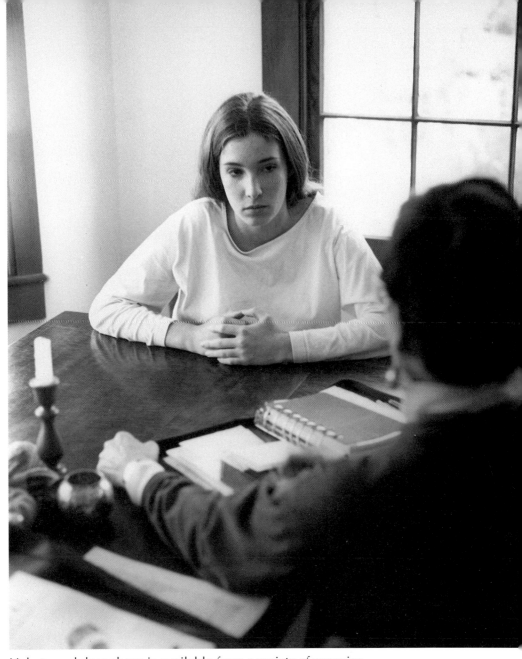

Help to end drug abuse is available from a variety of agencies and counselors.

The School Nurse

School nurses are trained to recognize and deal with medical problems like addiction. They can also help if you need emergency medical care.

The Police

The police may be the last people in the world that you want to tell about your drug abuse. But you can be sure that they know, or know how to find out, where to get help.

Certified Alcohol and Drug Counselor (CADC)

CADCs are *the* professionals in the drug and alcohol field. They can help you decide what steps to take to overcome your addiction.

To find a CADC, look in the Yellow Pages under "Alcoholism" or "Drug Counselors." You will find the letters CADC after the counselors' names. Call right away!

Your Doctor

If you (or a friend) have been using depressants for some time and then stop using for a day or two, you could go into withdrawal. *Call your doctor immediately* if you have any of the following symptoms: nausea, extreme nervousness, shakiness, stomach cramps, excessive sweating, convulsions, or delirium (seeing, hearing, or feeling things that are not there). You may need professional medical help.

Glossary
Explaining New Words

abuse Use of a drug in a manner other than that prescribed.

addiction State or condition of being unable to stop using a drug.

alcohol A depressant found in beer, wine, and liquors.

alcoholic Someone who is addicted to alcohol.

barbiturates Depressant drugs; they slow the mind and the body and kill in large doses.

cold turkey Suddenly stopping the use of a drug without medical help.

coma Unconsciousness.

convulsion Involuntary and violent spasm of the muscles.

depressant Drug that slows down the mind and body.

detox Process of stopping drug use.

dose Amount of a drug used at one time.

downer Slang for depressant. Some downers are alcohol, barbiturates, tranquilizers, and heroin.

drop To take a drug by mouth.

genetic tendency An inborn condition of being prone to something; in this book, being born prone to addiction.

60 **hypnotic** Drug that causes the user to go to sleep.

opium Depressant drug made from poppies.

speed Slang for a drug that excites the mind and body.

THIQ (tetrahydroisoquinalin) A chemical found in the brains of both alcoholics and cocaine addicts. It is believed to suppress the chemicals that give a sense of peace and well-being.

tranquilizer A class of legally prescribed depressants.

upper Slang for drugs that excite the mind and body.

withdrawal The physical effects of being without drugs.

HELP LIST

Alcoholics Anonymous World Services, Inc.
P.O. Box 459, Grand Central Station
New York, NY 10163

American Council for Drug Education
204 Monroe Street
Rockville, MD 20852
(301) 294-0600

Narcotics Anonymous World Service Office *61*
16155 Wyandotte Street
Van Nuys, CA 91406
(818) 780-3951

National Association of Children of Alcoholics
31706 Pacific Coast Highway
South Laguna, CA 95677
(713) 499-3889

National Clearinghouse for Alcohol and Drug Information
P.O. Box 2345
Rockville, MD 20852
(301) 468-2600

National Council on Alcoholism and Drug Dependency
12 West 21st Street
New York, NY 10010
(800) 662-HELP

National Federation for Drug-Free Youth
8730 Georgia Avenue
Silver Springs, MD 10910
(800) 554-5437

National Prevention Network
444 North Capitol Street, NW
Washington, D C 20001

For Further Reading

Ball, J. *Everything You Need to Know about Drug Abuse*, rev. ed. New York: Rosen Publishing Group, 1992.

Berger, G. *The Pressure to Take Drugs*. New York: Franklin Watts, 1990.

Black, C. *The Secret Everyone Knows*. Los Angeles: Operation Cork, 1981.

Clayton, L. *Amphetamines and Other Stimulants*. New York: Rosen Publishing Group, 1994.

_____. *Designer Drugs*. New York: Rosen Publishing Group, 1993.

Edwards, G. *Coping with Drug Abuse*, rev. ed. New York: Rosen Publishing Group , 1990.

_____. *Drugs on Your Street*. New York: Rosen Publishing Group, 1993.

Gravits, H., and Bowden, J. *Guide to Recovery*. Holms Beach, FL: Learning Publications, 1985.

Larson, E. *Old Patterns, New Truths*. New York: Harper/Hazelden, 1989.

Levy, S. *Managing the Drugs in Your Life*. New York: McGraw-Hill, 1983.

McFarland, R. *Coping with Substance Abuse*, rev. ed. New York: Rosen Publishing Group, 1990.

Smith, S. *Heroin*, rev. ed. New York: Rosen Publishing Group, 1993.

Index

About the Author
Dr. Lawrence Clayton earned his doctorate from Texas
Woman's University. He is an ordained minister and has
served as such since 1972. Dr. Clayton is a clinical mar-
riage and family therapist and certified drug and alcohol
counselor. He is also president of the Oklahoma Professional Drug and Alcohol Counselor's Certification Board.
Dr. Clayton lives with his wife, Cathy, and their three children in Piedmont, Oklahoma.

Photo Credits
Cover photo: Stuart Rabinowitz.
Photo on page 10: North Wind Picture Archives; all other
photos by Stuart Rabinowitz.

Design & Production: Blackbirch Graphics, Inc.